Brown Recluse Spider Bitten!

By

Martha Y. Wright C.F.Hom.

i

Publisher's Cataloging-in-Publication Data
provided by Five Rainbows Cataloging Services

Names: Wright, Martha Y., author.
Title: Brown recluse spider bitten! / Martha Y. Wright.
Description: Atascadero, CA : Wright Light Publications, 2018.
Identifiers: LCCN 2018911061 | ISBN 978-0-692-19009-8 (pbk.)
Subjects: LCSH: Brown recluse spider. | Spider bites. |
    Homeopathy. | Essences and essential oils--Therapeutic
    use. | Clay--Therapeutic use. | Women--Biography. |
    BISAC: BIOGRAPHY & AUTOBIOGRAPHY / Women. |
    BIOGRAPHY & AUTOBIOGRAPHY / Medical. |
    MEDICAL / Alternative & Complementary Medicine.
Classification: LCC RX66.W75 2018 (print) | LCC RX66.W75
    (ebook) | DDC 920.72--dc23.

Brown Recluse Spider Bitten!
Paperback @ 2018 by Martha Y. Wright C.F.Hom.
Wright Light Publications

Printed by KDP

Dedicated to the light that casts fear aside

CONTENTS

CONTENTS

Forward

This little book will mean a lot to those who have the dread of eight legged creatures. These fellow sufferers will have less fear once they know that they can deal with at least some of the legitimate concerns that all should really have for the arachnoids that we mutually inhabit the planet with.

While this book is a true account and shows how I dealt with a Brown Recluse Spider Bite successfully, it cannot possibly take the place of qualified and legitimate medical services. There are people with extreme sensitivities, weakened immune systems or the elderly, children, or perhaps diabetics that may need the extraordinary care offered by hospitals and medical doctors. A visit to websites that show photos of Brown Recluse bites and their aftermath show that the bite of this spider can be lethal or devastate lives.

Anyone seeking emergency care should go to an emergency center for help. However, the soonest I got help was many hours later, so it would behoove anyone to know how to handle this bite on an emergency basis by themself, if they cannot get help immediately. The bite is so painful that it is not practical to wait. In the end, the reader may get more out of this book, in the final analysis, than they will from many sources of medical services. The experience and treatment can add to the ability to deal with this very painful and even lethal bite. Also, it is certainly important to be prepared and to give close consideration to what is offered in this humble book. This book also would be of interest to medical doctors as a true case history. It should also be of interest to Homeopaths and Naturopathic doctors.

Brown Recluse Spider Bitten!

Chapter 1
The Background

An ancient wise man said, "Do you want to know other men? - know thyself. Would you like to know yourself? - then know other men." I am less philosophical and bluntly put, I say, "It takes one arachnophobic to know another arachnophobic." I won't say that I have had counseling or therapy for my condition. I won't say I was on tranquilizers or some other type of medication, but I lived with an awareness you must be cautious at all times indoors and out. Yes, be aware that a spider could appear at any time and most awfully - on a part of your body. You could never be too careful. They might drop down from a tree branch while you're innocently walking, or crawl up your pantleg. Indoors they might crawl out from under a couch cushion while you are relaxing watching a movie. Worst, they might attack you in the middle of the night, just when you think you're all snug and cozy, depriving you of that safe place in your life, that last refuge of security, when you're with your blankie. Maybe that's the real reason for that prayer:

> "Now I lay me down to sleep
> I pray the Lord my soul to keep"

(They didn't wear those lacey sleeping bonnets in bed in time's past or have canopy beds for nothing you know!) Perhaps it was a prayer voiced originally by an arachnophobic.

Perhaps spiders were created to let you know you are never really safe. I have managed to drift off to sleep only to have an image flash before my dream eyes, an image of a spider, and defying sleep's natural state of imposed paralysis, I bounded out of bed like a shot from a canon, quite sure that it was real. Now that is bad, but only a true arachnophobic would completely understand this.

Yes, I know psychiatrists provide very deep complex explanations for this condition/phobia. So, if I, instead of rolling my eyes, roll out the old files in the basement, I do remember my mother actually down in the basement ironing and talking about the "Tarantulas" with blue eyes, in the coal bin. I do remember being more concerned about why my mother seemed so unhappy and I said to her, "Mom why are you so sad." Was this the link? If it was, it is not a repeated common theme among others. I don't think this theory could stand up to scientific scrutiny. No, and I don't really remember being terrified. Nor was I obsessed with them at the time.

Then there was the other event. I was probably no more than three. It was a sunny day and I was, in my child-like fashion, sitting there with my bare legs stretched out and so inquisitive that I did not care about a Daddy Long Legs. I may have, at this time, never seen a spider before and the red alert light did not go on when I saw eight legs. I had no fear. Then it did it's little push up thing right on my leg and it bit me! I am sure it bit me and I screamed.

Years later, I was told by a neighbor who was an authority on these matters (as most neighbors are) that Daddy Long Legs are the most poisonous spiders in the world but their mouths are too small to bite.   I usually never question serious informants about the accuracy of their information. Why would anyone go spreading false information about spiders? The matter is far too serious. Oh yes, you may say, another urban legend, but have a care, urban legends are based on something. They just don't appear out of thin air. However, I know that it bit me. Perhaps it was my tender three year old skin that permitted it. I would say that spiders earn their reputation. This fear just does not come out of nowhere. I remember being totally unprejudiced about spiders up to this point.

No, but the great morbidity that became pathological? Well, it didn't start when we first moved to California from Ohio and were safe in a regular apartment building. It was after we moved to an old house. This old house was actually the church rectory of a Catholic Church. The Catholic church building was an arms-length distance from our house. It was there that my father actually paid a man to come out to the house just to kill a Black Widow Spider. I could see this was serious. You did not mess with them. I should add here that you did not mess with my father, and if my father had such a fear of them, I knew this was very serious. It was all over after that. They were terror itself!

Well, I later lived in far-away places. I was not completely certain, but in England, I thought, maybe they didn't have Black Widows there, so I felt safer. Still, never trust a spider, I said as I smashed a big English spider on my bedroom wall. It was only, after that violent act I was informed,"that spider lived there!" My decisive action was not taken well and was one more strike against me by my future Mother-in-law.

3

Later, when we lived in Canada in a big apartment building I never saw one. But we did go to "cottage country" and there were spiders there. Most strangely I once spent an entire night sleeping in the boat house after my new husband and I were exiled from the main cabin for making too much "noise" in the middle of the night. It was either that or a million mosquitos outside, with no shelter. As any Canadian knows, mosquitos and "Black Fly" flourish in the great vacation "cottage country" of Ontario. Most strangely I don't remember ever sleeping as well as I did in that boat house even aware that there were spiders right in that room. I will never understand that – ever. It was truly paradoxical.
Yes, there are strange things that go on in the complex minds of the arachnophobics. Things in the mind like flies caught hopelessly in the sticky web of creatures who, shall we say... have too many legs and move too fast.

Yes, this Jungian, paradox-like, primordial fear that preceeded my life, some would say, was a natural protective mechanism. Snakes, spiders, insects, it is a built in natural psychological mechanism that protects us from venomous creatures. Yeah, that is the logical explanation. The one that makes sense. You can try to reason with an arachnophobic on this basis but it will not stop them from screaming and literally running around in circles at the awful moment of confrontation, actually coming face to face with their nemesis. I know, I've been there.

Bi-annually I don the full gear of a hazardous waste costume of my own creation. It is make-shift, but it does the job. My pants are tucked into my socks. I wear rubber gloves, a hooded jacket, a mask and protective eye goggles as I spray and spray and spray, wherever I can outside to at least cause a decline in the population of the dreaded Black

Widow Spider. Just writing the name is enough to give me the "willys". I am so glad that they are really black. That way they are hard to miss. They stand out vividly, and if there is any doubt at all, you can turn them over and see the dreaded red hourglass.

There is a dismal and forbidden place, a closet in my car-port. It is a dark place, evil, and as I know very well, haunted by Black Widows. It is their full territory. I always walk as far away from the door as I can. I have been known to put on my full gear including a plastic bag over my head and bomb them.

In the ranch house, we unfortunately lived in, I came home one night and saw a huge, strange looking spider that had something weird on it's back. This was a time you did not ask questions though. It was time to "shoot first and ask questions later". In hind sight it may have been a "Recluse". You know I never had the desire to look at spiders in a book. It would make me nauseous. When I saw it, I took off my shoe in a flash and pounded it and pounded it till it was part of the floor all the while screaming to bring the house down. It was so strange, it had such a hard body. It just did not want to be flattened! We lived miles from anyone else or I would have had the neighbors breaking down the door. What it was, for sure, will never be known.

This brings up another important point. In spite of the paranoia intrinsic to arachnaphobia, it is an amazing observation that arachnaphobics will turn into killing machines at a moment's notice. Yes, they fear but they also kill! They will not suffer a spider to live. They will not allow them to crawl away and hide, and they certainly don't rescue them and put them outside so they can have a nice life. If these crazy people who rescue spiders thought about it, they just come right back in or attack you in the garden. No, they are dead meat! Speaking of dead meat, can you believe the Africans that eat those huge spiders? Like deep fry them. Death by starvation first, is what I say!

In this same ranch house I was ironing in the loft and suddenly a Black Widow was right in front of my eyes tangled in my hair. Yes, I went absolutely mad raving, screaming berserk. Clawing and hitting away like a maniac shrieking all the while. It is a wonder life went on in that house after that, if you know what I mean!

Many years later after an inevitable divorce, I was unpacking in my new little place and put my hand in a box and was immediately bitten. It was so viciously painful. I knew for sure it had to be a Black Widow. I screamed and literally ran around in circles in the kitchen. I thought, this is it, I'm a goner. Somehow, I got a hold of myself and thought to put ice on it. I then went to the phone to call my daughter to let her know I was going to the emergency and also possibly die, but the phone did not work! Why? I couldn't understand in my hysterical state. I then went to the neighbors and knocked on their door, trying to get help. No answer! I went back to my house and tried to use the phone. Nothing. I felt like I was slipping away. My thumb hurt so bad! I then went back to the neighbors and pounded on their door. No answer! I felt like I was in the twilight zone. I realized the only thing to do was for me to drive myself to the emergency. Would I make it? Would I have convulsions or die on the way? I made it there and called my daughter thinking it may be the last time I saw her. I saw the doctor and told my tale of woe. I had been bitten by a Black Widow after sticking my hand in a box, blindly, while unpacking. I had not been careful. Everyone sympathized. The doctor gave me anti-histamines and sent me home. That was it. All night I kept my hand in ice. Much to my surprise and relief, in the morning I saw what the real attacker was. There was a very large fat wasp in the sink. Somehow, I had killed the creature after it had stung me. I had not known really what was happening. It was all so strange as I had made arrangements with a bee sting therapist to have my hand stung because I was having some inflammation. The wasp had stung me in the exact spot that we would have chosen for the bee sting. I never had any more trouble with that thumb. It was not a bee, but the wasp worked. They say God works in mysterious ways (but this stretches even the most elastic mind). I have found this to be very true but also hard to take. No one said it would be easy. Right?

Many years later in a different place, I carefully sprayed and killed eighty Black Widows around my basement apartment in April. (That's the best time to find them outside) The next year only forty. The next year twenty and the last year ten. I cut their numbers in half every year. Although, I am pretty sure I did get bit by one in the long grass, getting groceries out of the car at night when I was wearing a skirt. Unaware of the bite at the time, it may have not been much of a bite, but I had a burning stomach for months after that bite. However, it was not the Black Widow that almost finished me off in that basement apartment. It was another unseen killer – mold!

It is a long story I will not go into depth about it, but yes, basement apartments and water leakage, and no ventilation. When I finally realized what was going on, I was almost finished. I fled that apartment as fast as I could and little did I know I would be facing the bite of an unexpected and unwanted invader on top of everything else! This, "move in great haste", is what led up to my encounter with the dreaded Brown Recluse.

Chapter Two
The "Bite"

By a miracle I got into another apartment. This one was far too expensive for me, but it was nicer. It was a town house with two bedrooms. It had a long flight of stairs up to the front door and a double flight of stairs inside. It had a lot of stairs. One would think too many stairs for even the most determined spiders. I managed to move all my "stuff" and was finally "stuffed" inside my new place with all my "stuff". "Stuff" that had sat in boxes in my old basement apartment in dark places. Whether I brought it with me or it was an inhabitant of my new dwelling, which was right on top of a very woodsy and wild creek, I do not know.

I even have the postulation that my former basement landlord put it in my jacket which had been in my car with the window down. He had definitely been sneaking around. He had come into my apartment when I was not there. His lingering cigarette smoke gave him away. I had called the police and the building department on him as I did not want anyone else to die from mold exposure like I was facing. He was not a nice man. In fact, he was the kind of person who would do something like that. Actually, if there is ever anyone writing on the most awful landlords of all time, he should be on the list.

Moving is hell and I was not in a good state. I should have given more awareness, after I moved, when my cat began acting strangely. It was, after all, our first night in a new place. You know how cats are. They totally freak out with moving and I had planned to keep him inside for at least two weeks after the move. You can expect some kind of strange behavior, but he was running up and down and up and down the new stairs in my apartment, all the while mewing to beat the band in the strangest tones – like me-Oowoww-ow ow ow oooow, over and over as he frantically ascended and descended. Up and down he went, not once or twice, but over and over. Even for a cat who is somewhat odder than most, and given to mad half hours, which very fairly regularly come on at ten o'clock at night, this was out of character. It was peculiar. Rather than listen to him, I scolded him. "What the (use your imagination) hell is wrong with you!", I shouted with great aggravation. If only I had realized what he was trying to tell me.

Of course the place was a mess, I had just moved in. I only managed to set up my bed for sleeping by the end of that long day. It was my first night in my new apartment. I woke to find blood on my sheet. This was highly unusual. In fact, it was a first. It was an unusual morning all in all as I would find out. Things were not going to go as planned. I barely had time to eat a hurried breakfast and get out the door to work. I jumped in my car and put on my jacket. It was then I felt a searing and brutal pain in my left elbow. I hastily took off my jacket. I strained to see that elbow area and was shocked to see, not a tack or a razor blade but two deep punctures on my left elbow. It was a spider bite! I was calm in the face of this crisis at first. It had happened, I had to face it. It was a spider bite and it was bad! I had never had a bite like this. I realized it was over, as far as work for that day. I immediately called the doctor's office and they could not see me till 5 o'clock! I would not make it that long. The pain was unreal. It was excruciating. In the face of real danger I am calm and fortunately, as time was of the essence, I thought of putting a clay pack on it. It was one of the best decisions I made in my life.

Chapter Three
Taking Action

After I realized I was not going to see a doctor till the end of the day and that the cost of another emergency room visit (after my "non" Black Widow bite $1,500 visit) was out of the question. It occurred to me to use a clay pack. I had used clay packs before for face packs and for bites. They have a wonderful effect for drawing out boils or just anything . I immediately made one up. I had always used what they call "French Clay" or one that was called "Aztec Clay". It is a little tricky mixing up these clays with water which I would like to explain later. I had, for years, incorporated a few drops of Essential Oils in the clay pack. This just quadrupled the wonderful effects with the drawing power of the clay. These oils were not just any Essential Oils – they were Young Living Essential Oils, which I had used for years in my massage therapy work. I had come to swear by them. I had seen such truly excellent results with them that I would never think of risking using anything else. I would not want to waste my time and take a chance on not getting results with very sick people who came to me for one problem or another. I will stop and say here that I eventually found the best oil to use for the bite of a Brown Recluse Spider is the combination essential oil that in the Young Living brand is called "Purification Oil". It is a combination which has Rosemary in it which is a powerful but gentle oil. Rosemary has anti-staphylococcus properties. I would like to tell you, here and now that using straight essential oils on an open wound is not a good idea. It would be too caustic. However, mixed in the clay pack it is fine. The clay pack was the best way and most powerful pain stopper. I was soon to be getting good experience with it all. Fortunately, I did it right the first time.

The proportions and way of mixing are as follows:
Put <u>two tablespoons of clay</u> (I use Aztec or French clay) into a small bowl. A large <u>custard cup rounded on the bottom</u> is best. Put in a <u>few drops of a plain oil</u>, I always use a cold extracted oil like Almond, Grapeseed, or Sunflower. Sprinkle <u>generous drops of your essential oil (Purification Oil</u> made by Young Living is the best) in as well. Add only about three tablespoons of plain water or better still Distilled Water. Add water at first all at once. The mixture is at first almost too thick to stir. Stir this thick mixture with a small stiff spatula or handle of the spoon. Thereafter, add 1 tbsp of water at a time, stirring after each addition of water. When you get the consistency that is usable and if you want to use it right away, then put on this thick, but plyable consistency. After putting a thick layer on the area, you can add several more tablespoon or so of water and stir again. Make sure you have a consistent smooth mixture. It will be thinner but will thicken up after sitting. Cover tightly. I have a container that has a tight lid that I use. Otherwise tightly wrap with plastic wrap and put a rubber band around it. It will dry out too much if you don't. Store in the refrigerator. It will feel really good cold.

After putting this clay pack on, immediately, the pain subsided. It was astounding. At first, I did not know what had bit me. My first thought was a Black Widow and that it had finally happened.

It is important to understand that spiders of any type can and most likely do carry Tetanus. Quite frankly just consider it a fact. They also carry other bacteria and parasites and I do believe, particularly, carry Staphylococcus. Rosemary and Olive leaf are effective against staphylococcus. I have even seen them get rid of the dreaded MRSA. I had long ago read that French hospitals used Rosemary to prevent staph infections in their hospitals.

There was a lot to do that day. It was hard to focus on anything else than the bite. It was a traumatic event for me. The clay was drawing but I observed in horror that the ulcer was still spreading going deeper and deeper still. I tried to distract myself, but I was worried. What would this mean? I knew that spider bites can cause a lot of other problems. They can cause ulcers in the blood vessels and the intestines. They can cause permanent arthritis. As far as I felt, they could cause insanity.

I did not know what type of spider this was. There was nothing to be done except face up to the fact that I had been bitten by the spider from hell which was still running around, lurking in my apartment ready to attack me at any moment. I could not have this. I went out and bought spider poison in a bottle to spray and I went over every area that was possible and began spraying. In most cases I am very much against spraying poisons. After all, I had a cat and did not want to spray where my dear cat might put a paw. Then I don't even like to use spays outside because of the birds, bees and butterflies. But for spiders I make an exception - I compromise . I have a middle of the road policy. I only use it or try to confine it to places where spiders frequent. This is on the edges of things and those dark places where they nest in their horrid webs. This time was the big exception. I must admit, I went a little crazy with the spraying.

Finally, it was time to go to the doctors. I was so relieved. I went to the office and then I had to wait another hour and a half in the waiting room! I was regretting that I had taken off my clay pack. I had done this because I wanted the doctor to be able to see the damage and also because I didn't want to be ridiculed by the doctor or get into "trouble" for putting on a clay pack. While I was there I watched a man who sat straight across from me.. I really did not have much choice but to observe him. The poor man was sitting there with his legs looking terribly enlarged, black and blue, and I could see, really, they were necrotic. I had taken care of such sad cases in hospitals. How did he get out into this terrible condition? Oh, the wonders of modern allopathic medicine! Just a little steroids and we'll keep you on those antibiotics. I was all too familiar with the pattern after working in hospitals and working for medical doctors in the allopathic field. I have seen the end results of steroids. I had experienced it's dark side years before and knew I would never trust it again.

As I sat there waiting, I was preparing myself for the battle that I always seem to get into with doctors. Not just this doctor, but all doctors for many years. I once had a doctor give me a totally free visit when I correctly diagnosed my son with thrush in the mouth. He then said, "No, he does not have thrush". I said, "Look again doctor!" . On the second examination he said, "Well I stand corrected and you are going to get a free visit!"! I say it's always a good idea to question your doctor but they don't like it much. So, look out! How I dreaded going to the doctors. Sometimes I would just get well while I was waiting. I would convince myself that I really didn't need to be here. But at this point I really needed the doctor. This was a clinic and I didn't know which doctor I was going to see. I had come in recently because of the mold issue but was not really familiar with the staff. Yes, the adrenalin was surging!

Then it seemed so suddenly that they called my name
and into the office I went - into the lions den! I had not seen
this doctor before. He was actually sympathetic . His first
words were, "That is the worst bite I have ever seen and that
is a Brown Recluse Spider bite!" He said this with a particular
note of horror in his voice. "I don't know how you can stand
the pain!" He looked at me in a type of way like wonder, and
I felt like saying, "You have no idea!" I wanted to tell him
about the clay pack and the Essential oils and how they had
instantly taken away the terrible pain, but I refrained.
He continued, "We don't have Brown Recluse in this area!
How could you get bit by one?" I just shrugged my
shoulders. "I have no idea. I have not even been out of the
county for a year. I did not see what kind of spider it was." I
did not argue with him but he spoke in a most insistent
manner saying that it was a Brown Recluse. "They don't
have to be very big. They can be very small and still do
that." "That" meaning this ulcer which was still growing and
deepening. He kind of gave a little shudder at the end and
then he said in a most emphatic way, "You will be in the
hospital on IV antibiotics by the weekend and we will most
likely", he stopped, "you will probably have to have that arm
amputated." That was pretty shocking . Secretly I blew that
off with a guffaw. Outwardly I just did not react. He said
again, "I don't know how you can stand the pain!". I tried to
look long suffering.

Then he said the magic words, "I'm going to give you a
prescription for an antibiotic." Thank God and thank
goodness!" I did not have to do battle with this doctor in
order to get a prescription for an antibiotic. I wish I could
have shared my valuable information about the clay pack
with him and the essential oils but I do not think he would
have been open to it. I would like to comment here that I had

15

read and researched information on Essential Oils for years and knew about University studies and tests that show: Essential Oils have powerful, anti-biotic, anti-viral and anti-fungal properties. I knew that whereas an anti-biotic may actually aggravate fungal and viral conditions, Essential Oils do not. They were really "broad spectrum." However, I really felt that an anti-biotic was essential too at this point. The condition was too severe to only rely on the Essential Oils. I did not want to take chances. I knew it was time to bring out the "big guns" and attack full force now before the condition got out of hand.

At this point my knowledge of homeopathy was limited. I had, back in 1990, been totally "cured" of Lyme Disease under the care of a homeopath. See my book, <u>Lyme Disease: How I Beat It</u>). I had also gotten rid of a singular outbreak of shingles when I was under severe stress with only homeopathy in only a few days. I knew it was beyond pointless to bring up homeopathy with a medical doctor. They are not trained in it at all and in fact are indoctrinated that it is ineffective and practically bordering on superstition, in spite of the fact that there are homeopathic medical doctors in this country and almost fifty percent of the world's doctors have training in homeopathy and do use it. Medical doctors, in training, in India must have three years of training in homeopathy.

I was still thankful for the empathy I received from this medical doctor and the prescription for one round of anti-biotics I received from him. Yes, I do appreciate medical doctors and the place they have in the medical world. I just wish they had more appreciation and understanding of homeopathy and did not engage in persecuting homeopaths along with their "big brother" pharmaceutical companies.

I left the office with prescription in hand. I would not say I left smiling but I immediately got the anti-biotic and started taking it according to directions. I felt much safer after receiving this prescription. I was very thankful for that doctor.

I asked if I should get a Tetanus shot, but he said no. In one way, I would say he was remiss but as I know now so much more about the dangers associated with Tetanus shots in particular, I am thankful that I did not get one.
I would like to insert here that there are remedies that are recorded in the Homeopathic Materia Medica as being effective in treating and prophylactically "getting ahead and stopping" Tetanus. Tetanus, like Rabies is such a terrible and fatal disease that I do not think I would like to take on a confirmed case of Tetanus without the care of a medical doctor being involved. However, you never know, homeopathy just might save the day!

There are several homeopathic remedies that have the case histories showing that they are effective against Tetanus and one is Hypericum. I will go more into Hypericum later.

As so often happens, the "amputation sentence" did not happen. Yes, I do realize that when a doctor speaks, when he says a patient has not long to live. When he says that this is a fatal disease, and you only have so many days or weeks, that people will die just simply as a result of this authority phenomenon. It is the "doctor as god" phenomenon. When the doctor speaks it very well may be the - "death sentence"! I have literally seen this happen several times. I have also heard of other people observing this same phenomenon. I wasn't so convinced. OK doctor we will just see about that! I thought it but I did not voice it;

I did not need to go on IV anti-biotics by the weekend. I did not have my arm amputated. If you think this was not a possibility, just peruse the internet for "images" of Brown Recluse Spider bites and take a look at people who had massive ulcers, massive inflammation and swelling. Actually, their arms or legs were rotting off their bodies. Painful? They were most likely on Morphine. Yes, amputations were done, life long problems no doubt followed.

Without going to great lengths to provide references, I can say that with my experience working in hospitals and for medical doctors, observing the case histories, using steroids, I would say that most of these hideous cases were expedited or exacerbated by originally taking steroids! <u>Steroids softens tissues increasing and spreading any infection already in the body</u>. I think steroids should be used only in life threatening emergencies and where there is no alternative.

I have seen several cases where doctors gave shots for pain of unknown origin, only to find that the patient had Valley Fever. I did not know, at the time, that Valley Fever could spread it's tentacles out under the influence of steroids. In these cases, it did not confine itself to the lung cavity but filled the abdomen and rotted the spine out. One man had PVC pipe supporting his spine after this terrible "side effect" of this much used tactic of allopathic medical care. No doubt it severely shortened his life.

The main problem with the bite of this dangerous spider is not only the poisonous venom, but also the disease germs that the spider is carrying. Steroids tends to spread the infection.

Thankfully, I did not have to see that doctor again because by the weekend I was not in the hospital on IV antibiotics, nor was I facing the unthinkable – amputation, but I was instead, making headway against this horrific bite.   Yes, the antibiotic and also the clay pack with the "Purification" Essential Oil blend in it did start a healing process.

Chapter 4
Paranoia Set In

Yes, I did start on my anti-biotic and continued with the Purification Oil in the clay packs. I was glad that something worked but the dread of this spider lurking around in my large apartment was overpowering my good sense. I continued looking for it and spraying.

When I got home, I took all the covers off my bed, in fact, I stripped it down to the mattress and moved the mattress off the bed. I looked underneath. It could have been hiding under my mattress - some how. I forgot to mention in one place I did find a Black Widow nesting between the mattress and the mattress pad corner! What a shock that was.

Later I had, and still have, a client who was bitten by a Black Widow in bed. It is worth telling the story now. She was sleeping in bed with her husband and she felt she must have had her hand outside the covers. I mention this because there is some fear amongst some of us that you just don't let your hands or arms out over the covers at night in bed. So great and common is the fear that putting one's hand down over the edge of the bed, has been the subject of late night talk shows. In fact, I have heard some say that it goes back to that old primordial fear, the twin of which is monsters under the bed or in the closet. At any rate she awoke with excruciating pain. She said she knew it must have been a spider. Her husband rushed her to the emergency and she was in terrible stomach pain. Rather than listen to her explanation for her pain, the doctors wanted to do exploratory surgery. Strangely, one nurse, must have believed her, and refused to cooperate. In the meantime, her husband rushed home to look for the Black Widow. 33Amazingly, he found it and brought it back in a jar. This ba3rely saved her from exploratory surgery. She recounts that in the next days she was hospitalized, she was in agony and nothing they did helped. Strange things later happened to her. She developed severe and permanent, very disfiguring, Vitiligo. (This is when the skin loses it's pigment in patches). I researched this and found that the Pituitary has some play in this. I wondered, as I researched her homeopathic case, did Black Widow venom affect the pituitary? Later arthritis became a terrible problem in her life. Yes, arthritis can follow spider bites.

So yes, the fact is the bed was the first place I scouted. The thought came, though, I do not want the bed next to the wall. I moved many boxes and put the bed in the middle of the room. I left off any sheets and decided to sleep with just a heating blanket over me. That's it - give it no place to hide. I started straightening a few things up and kept looking in expectancy that a spider could jump me at any moment or be crawling around on the floor. That was the first night's pre-sleep fear.

I lay awake for hours in dread. Suddenly I woke up in the night and jumped out of bed. I was sure the spider was out now waiting to attack in the dark. I ran for the light switch. I looked around the room. My heart pounding. I tore off the blanket. I looked under the bed. I looked all around the room. Yes, that may be somewhat normal- but I did it several times more in the night. It became the pattern. I quickly became sleep deprived

I was no stranger to sleep deprivation, but this was especially bad. As soon as I went to sleep it seemed I was waking, with shock and jumping out of bed. I decided to just sleep with the light on. After all, the spider had to be dissuaded from attacking me!

Although I was feeling that, for the most part, the open ragged ulcer was being kept at bay, I almost returned to the doctor for more anti-biotics. The bite was still extremely painful. The only thing that helped it was the clay pack. However, like many people, anti-biotics make me so sick. I decided to stick it out a little longer.

As I mentioned, I had such a terrible time with my landlord before I left my basement apartment. I had indeed turned him into the building department. I had though, managed to get my rent deposit back. This was not what usually happened with him. He had bragged to me before, that people did not leave his premises without paying thousands of dollars for things that he considered that they had damaged. He and his wife had actually sued her mother in court and their only daughter as well. I did an immaculate cleaning job and spent an entire day cleaning the apartment. Meanwhile, I also took photos of mold under things and documented everything. I wasn't sure how things would worK out but I typed single spaced, six pages of history recounting the last four years of abuse by him and his wife and let them know I was going to get my deposit back! By the way, it did work!. However, the second day after I moved in I came back to my new apartment to find some strange wire clippings and electrical parts on my doorstep. In my paranoia and sleep deprivation, I somehow imagined that he had put a bomb somewhere like when I would open the door. I went and found a military man I knew and asked him what I should do. He must have thought me crazy. To this day I do not know what the wires etc. were, that were on my doorstep.

I think that this nightmare landlord really left them there to scare me. A few years later I found out he went to prison for selling Heroin. As I said, a dangerous man, a bully and quite possibly a person who would go to any lengths to get revenge. I knew this and in my paranoid mental state I really did see it that way.

I began to see, not only paranoia was a prominent feature of this particular spider bite, but it was getting the better of me. I needed something more to take care of myself.

Yesterday I was invited to a barbecue and mentioned this book. As it turned out the host had been bitten by a Brown recluse. He talked about the pain and that it caused a huge painful abscess at the site of the bite which was at the back of his head. He endured it for two days and then went to the emergency. The good doctor drained it and he went on antibiotics. It helped but he seemed to get some infections after that including in his ear near the bite. He also said his perspiration smelled strange and strong after that for a long time. When he went out of the room his wife said that he became really paranoid after the bite. I was quite intrigued by this and suggested it may be good for him to do a course of the next remedy I took which follows.

Chapter Five
Something More

Yes, something more was needed. At this point in my life I had very little experience with homeopathy. All I knew was that it worked like nothing else did. You see, I had actually had full blown Lyme Disease and been cured of it around 1990. I kept intending to make a study of it, but over the years, I had only obtained a copy of Boericke's Materia Medica and that was all. I had no idea of what a Repertory was or how to use it.

AGARICUS MUSCARIS

However, while I was somewhat lost I did manage to actually get a few good remedies right. With my slim experience I managed to notice that I was getting twitchings on opposite sides of my body and actually more than that -like left arm and right foot. The remedy that came up was Agaricus. I read up on this very interesting remedy. It was associated with great fear but also, shall I call it a kind of blind, insane, crazy bravery. Agaricus was what the Vikings took that made them go "Berserker". Yes, they took it full strength in the mushroom form, in an allopathic or gross, large dose. Agaricus had this effect and it could, of course, be lethal. But in homeopathy, the curative side is seen in all poisonous plants and is captured by the homeopathic pharmacy. So as "like cures like", it was obviously what I needed. It would work in "reverse" to cancel out the paranoia. I had paranoia and I had the most characteristic kind of twitchings from one opposite side to the other but also not only that it was left elbow, right leg. Agaricus also has insomnia that is characterized by not being able to fall asleep while one is in expectation of being disturbed. I certainly had that as well.

BELLADONNA & CALCAREA CARBONICA

It's hard looking back to realize, I also managed to find and use Calcarea Carbonica. That was not so easy to figure out. Amazingly it did help with everything. I could not understand why as I knew it was just calcium – carbonized calcium. Years before this bite in 2007, I had been totally cured of Lyme Disease in 1991. I know that the word "cure" is not allowed in some circles of medicine. All I can say is that the very bad symptoms of that disease were completely removed by a course of Belladonna. Eight months of one 15 c Belladonna. After that course, I never experienced the same terrible symptoms of Lyme Disease again. They did not return. Years later, in 2010, when I began to study professionally I did understand why and I will not keep you in suspense about it. As I later learned, Belladonna is an acute of Calcarea Carbonica. I knew nothing of the concept of constitutional remedies or constitutional prescribing. Calcarea is still a good remedy for me. I am evidently a Calcarea by birth.

In years after 1991 I had used Belladonna a few times. I had used it for spider bites as I recognized with certain bites that the pain followed the nerves. Yes, the toxins actually travel up the nervous system and follow it. Belladonna works powerfully on the nervous system. It especially relaxes the parasympathetic nervous system. It just "flips that switch" somehow and relaxes you when you can't relax. It does not "drug" you. Like all homeopathics it just removes the undesired symptoms. I would like to say here and now that it is no wonder that Belladonna is such a wonderful healer. All healing takes place when the body is sleeping. When it is at rest. It is a beta blocker and an anti-inflammatory, and lowers fevers. Belladonna has a record of being the best remedy to use in certain epidemics with fevers. It has saved thousands of lives in the last two centuries. Belladonna has a peculiar type of insomnia that I had much of my life. A person believes he/she is awake and yet someone else will say he/she was sleeping. It has an annoying and exhausting quality of being unable to get fully asleep.

GUACO

I had also found out that Guaco is also a good one for spider bites. I had been bitten by spiders a few times in my basement apartment and they were what they call "Sun Spiders". I would wake up with my left leg jerking. What a pain they are! Spiders that is!

It seems though that this Brown Recluse required something else. I read that they have been studied and that victims also have ulcers in the blood vessels and intestines. That was the thing, I really did not feel too good. Was this a result of this "poison" spreading? Was this going to develop into something else?

HYPERICUM

In the meantime. I also read about Hypericum. Hypericum is a big remedy for bites. It is effective against Tetanus. I will say here and now that Tetanus is nothing to mess around with. It is a very serious and mostly fatal infection and I will add here an extremely painful way to go. A nurse once told me that she took care of a person with Tetanus and if a door was slammed down the hallway or any loud noise, it would send the patient into convulsions. Even so this doctor had not thought it necessary to give me a Tetanus shot. I felt better taking the Hypericum. It really did help noticeably with the pain. If you ever expect you have Tetanus seek attention from a medical doctor. However, you may also try Hypericum in conjunction with this. I would like to add that although Tetanus is in the dirt and you don't need to "step on a rusty nail" to get it, I do know of a case, 100% for sure, of a woman who got Tetanus at the dentist. She did survive but was extremely emaciated after the ordeal. Remember Tetanus is also known as "Lockjaw". She could not eat for a long time and was in the hospital for about two months. They did track it down to the dentist.

SUMMARY

So, as it turned out, I found most of my help and relief with homeopathic remedies: Belladonna, Agaricus, Calcarea Carbonica, and Hypericum.

All remedies were in about 30 c potency. It is important for you to understand that with homeopathy, less is better. A 30c is usually taken, at the most twice a day. It is not that it is dangerous, it is that you will desensitize yourself to the action of the remedy and it will not work. Homeopathics trigger your own body's immune response. You don't want to stop that mechanism. The first three days you should be able to take a remedy in 30 c, three times a day for 3 days but then cut down to 2 and in a week, most likely, just one a day. It is best to see a Homeopath for guidance but you might take it a long time at farther intervals of time. There are also LM potencies which are prepared a little differently and are preferrred by many homeopaths now. The clay pack with Purification oil in it, was an absolute life saver.

Chapter Six
The Encounter

In spite of my sickish state and the pain in my left elbow, I was working. I was thankful it was not my right arm that was bitten. The pain was extreme at times when the clay pack dried out. Did I mention that? Yes, it pretty much has to be moist to be drawing or effective.

Oh, I was working alright. Also, it takes me months to get organized after moving. It is what I call "moving hell". I was no stranger to moving. My parents had moved many times and guess who did the work. Although of tender years, as my mother worked, I was the one that packed, precleaned the new place, unpacked and cleaned up the old place. I had moved so many times that I really had a dread of it. What an ordeal it was!

This time though I had really added to it as I had bought a couple of book cases and a table and was finishing them in an Antique Ivory Crackle - no less. I had no experience in doing crackle and I wanted it to be perfect. More than that - they had to dry. So, many boxes were stacked and covered my living room floor. It was still a mess everywhere. I was still in a semi-paranoid alert state.

It had been two weeks since the bite and I came home after working all day. It was later than usual and my apartment had been dark and quiet all day. I walked in and turned on the light. Did I see something moving on the floor in the living room between all those books stacked? Yes I did! It was sudden and although I was in a kind of shock, all I could think was no! I cannot let it get away! Oh No! It was not going to get away and continue to sneak around and keep me living in dread and suspense. I had to be quick. I had no time to find something to hit it with. In an instant I grabbed the only thing I could - just a piece of paper. I would have liked it to be at least a shoe but as it was too fast and was making straight for the book pile a few inches away I saw in horror that this <u>was</u> the one. I saw, in a flash, the big fiddle on it's back and I smacked it again and again. God how I hated that popping feel as I crushed it's body under my hand with nothing but a thin piece of paper between me and it's disgusting body! I screamed and screamed and hit it and hit it. I was all the while thinking that I really should put it in a jar. Too late for that. It was a smear – that's all. Just a smear of spider guts! Ugh! Ooh ooh. Only an arachnophobic would understand!

Although a sense of triumph filled me after this horrific encounter, although I felt somewhat relieved, when it was over, I tried to push the thought back – Is this the only one?

I began telling everyone my story. The librarian informed me that they have to be careful when they get books out of the book drop. They have encountered Brown Recluse Spiders in there. The library was about a mile or less from my apartment. It is actually quite aways from the creek. I, on the other hand, was virtually on top of a very woodsy area and the creek. Well so much for there being no Brown Recluse Spiders in this area, doctor. Does this not bring to my mind the other doctor years ago that told me that there was no Lyme Disease in this area? Oh Sigh! Sigh..sigh!

Chapter Seven
The Battle Continues

After the initial encounter with the enemy and it's merciless attack, the remains of it's poisonous venom and the thought of it's filthy fangs dripping with staphylococcus or parasites or whatever, the effects lingered in skirmishes that lasted a year.

It took three months for the deep ulcer about the size of a quarter, went through to the muscle tissue, to finally start minimizing and settle into a scar that is about the size of a dime. It is a scar that is still quite visible.

I am a huge believer in Epsom Salts. This is one thing I have not shared to this point. I alternated putting Epsom Salt dilutions on this wound. Epsom Salts draws out poisons. It is really Magnesium Sulphate. (I actually worked at Epsom District Hospital in Surrey, England) So, by alternating I kept the scab from forming and blocking off the clay and it's healing properties, as well as the benefits of the salt. I wanted it to heal from the deep to the surface - from the inside to the out. Not to scab over or just heal on the surface. I have always done this. I have always known this. It is so important to understand this. Doesn't that make sense? Do you understand what I am saying?

For a couple of years I still felt sharp pains and aching pains in my elbow and muscles. The muscles in the area of the bite were weak. I still had twitchings. I still had symptoms. For this I found Hypericum worked best for the pain and Agaricus for the twitchings. That is why it is so important to carry on in a symptomatic way to eradicate the entire picture of this dreaded bite. It really is quite a deadly and bad spider. I don't take spider bites for granted and neither should you.

I had several people say quite seriously, "You had better not ever get bitten by that spider again!". Like no kidding! I had no intention of it. I took precautions like you wouldn't believe as I really did not want to get bitten again. One lady said, "You could die." Yeah, I already figured that one out! Yes, it is quite a burden, in many habitations to keep them at bay. I see now in the hardware store they have spider traps. I am not sure how well they work but I do believe in screens, spraying, and moving furniture and cleaning all areas of your place regularly. Yes, I have found Black Widows. I wish I lived in a more secure area. Some people though may not be so careful and bring them in, hiding in wood or furniture or whatever. They need to think again and be more careful. These biters are real and a literal pain to deal with.

The after affects of Brown Recluse can linger, that is, if you survive, without amputation or other diseases that they bless you with. Like I said, check out the internet images of Brown Recluse.

No doubt some were made worse by being given sterioids of one type or the other. I have been truly blessed to have learned the healing methods of homeopathy that has spared me considerable pain and disease.

Chapter Eight
Finding Peace

Homeopathy and the experience I went through actually helped me immensely to overcome my fear of spiders. Now, I knew I could deal with bites and the paranoia successfully. Yes, this was a big thing in my life. Now I know I can deal with spiders. I may not like them now, but I at least feel that I have some control over the situation if I am so unfortunate as to be bitten again.

I have played up this story, a little for humors sake, but really it is ironic that the experience strengthened me. You know there is a South American saying, "What doesn't kill you makes you stronger." This is quite like Homeopathy! It is the blessing of homeopathy that really made the difference. For one thing I know that the bite and it's effects can be overcome with Homeopathy even more so than Allopathic medicine. This is a great comfort. Homeopathy is the answer to so many toxins and poisons that we face in this world.

To utilize homeopathy at it's best, you must deal with things immediately. Yes, the sooner the better! Homeopathy is a vibrational medicine. It is smart to assess what is going on in the body before damage to organs sets in. Think of it as being like a physical to check out everything when you are not sick. There are telltale signs and warnings throughout the body that tell where trouble is developing. <u>There are patterns that display constitutional remedy needs. Some things do not seem to be so serious, but trouble starts displaying in symptoms and patterns of symptoms.</u>

However, there are many cases where there has been damage and homeopathic remedies have corrected these damages. Also, a different approach can be used. After all, once a disease sets in you have a different situation, a different remedy picture presents itself.

One example is a person who has developed bone spurs or other issues with calcium deposits. This may have been prevented, in the first place by the person taking not only minerals but the homeopathic form of the minerals. This is when there is an assimilation issue that is on a cellular level. The homeopathic form of the mineral works to help the body to assimilate the deficient mineral. The fact is some people can take a lot of calcium or whatever mineral and they just simply are not absorbing it. The homeopathic form of the minerals actually "trains" your body to accept the mineral. The longer you wait, the less likely you will be able to use only homeopathic remedies. To be sure, you can still benefit, but the longer you wait, the longer it will take for the remedy to work.

Here is another example. This is true of snake bites, bee stings, wasp stings and things like Poison Oak. Everyone knows that if one is bitten by a snake, it is crucial to get the anti-venom as fast as possible. Yes, people may later take antibiotics or other drugs but the only way to stop the action of the poison is with anti-venom. This is an Isopathic principle - almost homeopathic. Homeopathy uses a "similar" remedy.

I have used Poison Oak homeopathically prepared to stop the action of getting Poison Oak, with great success for myself. Other people may not find Poison Oak their remedy. They may need another remedy like Anacardium (which is related to Poison Oak) or some other remedy. Taking Poison Oak Remedy will actually stop some people from getting it even if they are exposed, if they take it before exposure.   Taking it prophylactically has worked for me.

It is best to work with a homeopath before you get into an emergency situation. Having a good casetaking and getting all possible information on a person may make a big difference if there is an emergency later. I do extremely detailed cases and notations in all my patients.

Chapter Nine
Lingering Effects

Although it took about three months for the gaping ragged wound to close, there were twinges of symptoms that haunt me still. The scar remains to this day – ten years ago now, a scar the size of a dime on my left elbow.

HYPERICUM

Yes, for years, I would suddenly feel pain and achiness in the area of the bite. I found Hypericum would, in this case stop this peculiar sensation and no doubt does good.

LEDUM PALUSTRE & BELLADONNA

A good remedy to keep on hand in your home pharmacy for bites is Ledum Palustre, especially spider bites. It has also been used for Lyme disease. I am not sure it would be completely effective against Lyme Disease. You may need another remedy. If you know you are bitten, I would certainly recommend going to a medical doctor as well as taking the Ledum Palustre. This would be something to use immediately after a bite, or soon thereafter. I did, in fact, get re-bitten by a Lyme tic after I was cured and of course I was very upset. (Lyme tics are so small. They are no bigger than the period at the end of a senctence.) I immediately started a course of the Ledum Palustre and did not have a recurrence of what I had been through before. If you have been bitten by a tic I would definitely ask your doctor to go on a course of antibiotics but I would also use the Ledum Palustre. It would not hurt to follow up for a period of time with the Ledum Palustre.

I would use the Ledum Palustre first for spider bites to start with. If it does not work enough, if the pain is traveling the nerves - think of Belladonna.

A homeopath can also help you get over the bad side effects of antibiotics. When I worked for a doctor of Internal Medicine, we used to give people "Bacid". Why do they not do that now?

ARSENICUM ALBUM

If I had already been through my Homeopathic studies I would, no doubt, have used Arsenicum Album. This can be used for ragged ulcers and the burning pain associated with the bite of the Brown Recluse Spider. These symptoms are an indication for Arsenicum Album. Remember it also has pathogens in it's bite.

I would also like to pass along to the reader now, that Arsenicum is one of the most effective things you can take for food poisoning that's origin is bad meat. You will be positively amazed at it's effectiveness. I had a client who had been on many antibiotics for an intestinal diarrhea that simply would not go away. One cost $1,200.00. I gave her one Arsenicum Album and this stopped the diarrhea and it did not come back. She had become so emaciated she looked like a concentration camp victim. She recovered after months of other treatments. I was amazed at the results myself!

Another excellent remedy for some bites is the Homeopathic remedy called Guaco. I found it particularly effective against what is called "SunSpiders" which had bit me in my bed. I knew I had been bitten because my <u>left leg would start jerking</u>. Sure enough, there was a bite. Darn those spiders!

Chapter Ten
Not Totally Negative

There is one outstanding story I have heard of and I am typing out a link source for the net. The link may not work in the future, but at the moment, this is it:

http://geekologie.com/2009/03/real-life-spiderman-paralyzed.php

The story revolves around a man who was paralyzed to some degree in an accident and actually it was quite serious as it appeared to be permanent. It seems he benefitted from the bite of a Brown Recluse Spider as it countered the paralysis in a "like cures like" fashion. In this case the spider prepared the correct potency and dose for the man.

This is quite possible homeopathically speaking. Homeopathy uses all kinds of venomous creature remedies in a beneficial way. It even uses Black Widow venom – Latrodectus mactans or "jaws of death". It is not a standard remedy but should only be used by skilled homeopaths. It is used for myocardial infarction and angina pectoris. Yes, it has a strong effect on the heart and used for extreme pain in that area. Considering the homeopathic concept of the "doctrine of signatures" is it not amazing that the Black Widow has a red hour glass on its abdomen.

Never try to make your own remedies of very poisonous things like this. Also, do not be considering a remedy like this for self prescribing. It has a complete profile and requires a skilled professional to use it.

This is a good time to bring up what has become my belief based on much study and observation of so many facts of homeopathy, science and study of nature. *I have come to see that all poisonous plants and animal venoms were designed by the Great Designer to be used as healing agents when prepared in a homeopathic form.* In a standard allopathic pharmacy they would be quite deadly but prepared according to homeopathic pharmacy they can have almost magical healing powers. *This, to me, proves homeopathy to be of divine origin.* It is the original way that these great healing substances were to be prepared as medicines. Yes, some things can be taken in a traditional herbal form, such as things that are of traditional use and not so toxic. However, very poisonous things prepared in homeopathic pharmacy can cure more dire conditions. In "gross" allopathic dosage they would kill. Yes, I say, why would there be so many poisonous substances designed for this earth if in fact not for healing purposes? Of course, some things could be used for insecticides.

Now may be the right time to introduce you to some basics about homeopathy. How does it work? It is necessary to understand some basics about disease and related subjects to do so .

Chapter Eleven
What is Homeopathy and How Does It Work?

I would like to give, as briefly as possible, an overall portrait of what homeopathy is about and how it works. I would like to counter some of what the critics of homeopathy are espousing. I would also like to explain some of what I can also reasonably follow through with an understanding of how homeopathy must work, because all is not completely understood.

There are many things we and even scientists use today, but as my grandfather who was a scientist and inventor said, "We don't understand it – we just use it". Yes, my grandfather, James Gillespie Allen, invented a type of vacuum tube for the radio. He also worked for General Electric and invented many things. I know he went to Carnegie Tech in the early years of the 20th century and was a scholar and a gentleman but besides the above quote which my mother passed on to me I know little. He always brought me books to read and once a pair of binoculars to help me in my star gazing. Yes, there are many aspects of science that we use and really, little is fully understood. We, in effect, just know enough to "use them".

Many medical doctors around the world receive homeopathic training. In India medical doctors must take three years of Homeopathic training to obtain their medical degree. In Germany, England and throughout Europe homeopathy is taught in medical schools and is used regularly by many people to good success. The Royal Family of Britain has been a great supporter of homeopathy for generations. Prince Charles has been an outspoken advocate.

Many don't understand what homeopathy is. They think it is "home medicine". Let me set the record straight on this. Homeopathy is not home medicine but derives from the words - "Like cures like". Rather than being home medicine whipped up in the kitchen, it is a highly sophisticated science that requires many years of study based on hundreds of thousands of man hours of research and meticulous observation of "trials" or what homeopathy calls "provings" of remedies on thousands of people or "provers". Sound familiar? Homeopathy was ahead of it's time in clinical drug tests. Homeopathic remedies have been given much more study than today's clinical drug trials and many have been used in that homeopathic form for the last two hundred years. Unlike many allopathic drugs, they have not caused deaths or been recalled due to causing injuries. Also, unlike "big Pharma" today, it was not all about trillions of dollars of profits.

Many wonder why cannot both be used and why can't they kind of "merge"? Homeopathy and allopathy seem to have opposing viewpoints. In many aspects homeopathy and allopathy seem to be enemies, that they are diametrically opposed in their philosophies and practice. This does not have to be 100% eternally true as both are a form of medicine. It is important to know when and how to bring each method into the forefront of the complexities of the healing process.

Let me stop here and just mention that word healing or cure. It is not allowed. Yet, it does happen. It certainly does happen in homeopathy. I was cured of Lyme Dsease. Yes, cured and I feel quite free to say that. (See my book: Lyme Disease: How I beat It. For those who want to make years of study, it is really desirable that allopathy should be a last resort or for those who have proven to be too far advanced in their disease state to be helped with homeopathy.

Also, in extreme medical emergencies allopathic procedures can be best, but sadly, not always. Emergency physicians are not trained in emergency homeopathic care and most homeopaths are not experienced enough with full medical knowledge and training to take on severe medical emergency care. They would also have to be able to switch to allopathic methods in a moment's notice if it was needed. With the exception of the few medical doctors in this country, who are also trained extensively in homeopathy, few would do it even if it was allowed. The fact is physicians must follow many rules that are accepted medical practice for medical doctors and they would be in serious trouble if they altered their protocols of treatment. That there are standards has proved a safeguard in some respects. Unfortunately, it has also assured that people never know or understand the superiority and validity of homeopathic philosophy and treatment. Medicine like life is full of paradoxes.

So what is the difference between allopathic medicine and homeopathic medicine? It is necessary for many people to learn that the medicine which is practiced by medical doctors and which they are mostly familiar with is called "allopathic" medicine. It is a system of suppression of symptoms.

Homeopathy differs from allopathic medicine in:

#1 it's theory
#2 it's pharmacy
#3 it's practice
#4 it's regulation
#5 it's results

It is necessary for many to understand what is so different about the approach of medicine used by what we call medical doctors and homeopathy.

Firstly, the differences have been going on for a long time. I can not be going into depth on this history, as it would be volumes, but we can see from the ancient records of Egyptian, Greek and Roman medical manuals there began a divergence in opinion of the overall approach as to how to handle medical care. What later became a more homeopathic approach began with more attention to observation and attention to individualizing care as to the particular differences observed in patients with regards to their temperament, their body types and what they did when they got sick. There also seems to be some recognition of "like cures like", even immunizations, and a "doctrine of signatures" in herbalism. Later, this type of doctor, epitomized by Samuel Hahnemann as he became prominent by use of the scientific methods of observation, progressed to a highly refined state and became the foundation of homeopathic practice. Hahnemann, a medical doctor of his day at the end of the 1700's, began the modern pharmacy of Homeopathic Practice.

To return to history, the face of allopathy was much about having set protocols for disease and treating disease as a mostly outside force. The concept of poison it, burn it, or cut it out is still very much the standard in the allopathic approach. In allopathy, along with set protocols there is much to be presumed as a result of studies that look to override the body's mechanisms and force the body, by means of strong drugs or poisons to do so. Even just cut it out if it doesn't do what you want it to! My observation has also seen that doctors want to see and look to diagnose according to preconceived sets of diagnostics. How many times have I seen that they do not take the time to carefully examine a patient, or even touch a patient. Today, in our litigatious society, touching seems to be even more taboo and that their main concern is to avoid being sued! If I was the only one who had this observation I could be challenged but it is widely recognized by many people I have talked to.

Although a homeopath can do a good consultation over the phone or Skype, they will be interested in every detail. If you have a pain it will need to be described in detail. Is it burning, stitching, tearing, pounding lancinating, prickling, hot, cold or any other description? Does the pain extend? What time of day is it worst or better? What different things affect it? In fact an extensive case history is in order that would include the entire person's history as well as his/her mother and father and other relatives. The entire person including mental and emotional is considered "in totality".

Homeopaths call allopathic drugs "gross" in that they have not been prepared by homeopathic pharmacy. These allopathic drugs can kill or cause much damage. That is why it is necessary to have a doctor's prescription. Many over the counter drugs are also allopathic and can kill. An example is Ibuprofen, Aspirin and Tylenol. Indeed the number of deaths induced by allopathic drugs, whether by prescription or over-the-counter in the United States alone each year, is in the hundreds of thousands. I am not even talking about street drugs which are also in the "gross" allopathic form.

Homeopathic remedies are different in that they do not over-ride the body but only stimulate the body's natural healing defense system. They "teach" the body.

I and other Homeopaths follow evidence that the homeopathic remedy communicates with the cells in the body in the body's own "language". A language involving, whether photons of light or on the ionic level, or simply magnetic, it is still debated. Now we are getting into some theory, but it has been given enough evidence to my satisfaction. There is no way that homeopathy could work as it does if it did not have the ability to change the body on a cellular level. Do you think that erroneous? Viruses in our body do it all the time. They commandeer the cells and make them produce toxins. Yes, viruses commandeer cells and make them replicate copies of the virus as well as toxins. They take them over. Now how do they do this? I cannot explain that now but we know that they do.

My big breakthrough in seeing this was when I first studied the disease of Syphilis. Syphilis is caused by a spirochete. It is important to understand that spirochetes have characteristics of both a virus and a bacteria.

I realized myself that the homeopathic form of the substance has to have the ability to change or at least cure the pattern at the deepest cellular level. Whether it is in the DNA, the RNA or the damaged mitochondria, it had corrective or restorative effects and overcame the disease which is entrenched at the cellular level. Yes, Syphilis has the ability to damage the very basic part of the cell. I would like to think of it as the DNA but whether it be that or the mysteries of magnetic mitochondria in the cell, it is not like many diseases. It is progressive, it hides out, it reappears, it digs in and continues to actually alter the cell. It has stages. That Syphilis was arrested and can be erased by homeopathic remedies is amazing and tells us much about it's potential. When I first read this I knew I was on to something regarding the DNA, but I found out later that medical doctors who were homeopaths had already figured this out. Remember, at the time, Samuel Hahnemann did not know about DNA, or in matter of fact, the proven existence of microbes. That was very soon to change though. He did however, by deduction, guess or know that something like that was going on!

I should insert here that homeopathic preparation of remedies helps the body when it is stuck or has "forgotten" it's own programming. This was later confirmed as I heard medical doctors who were homeopaths say the same thing. Yes, they too could see that homeopathy has the ability to re-alter, as it were, the DNA or ?. It had to be able to do it to have effect on such diseases like Syphilis. Is there any way of proving this now? Surely by the absence of the disease and yet also by scientific studies. There is much that I choose not to cover in detail right now in this humble little book.

Science in the field of industry and chemistry has discovered that succussing and diluting water many times changes water and this process has the ability to "reverse" or make a mirror image of molecules. The scientists in these fields were not trying to support homeopathic theory. Some did realize it did though and made it known. <u>This is exactly what had been suspected by Homeopaths since Hahnemann said that the remedy could cancel the disease by an opposite and equal force basically of the same pattern and also force of strength, making a reverse image.!!!</u> Water itself is an amazing substance which is taken for granted all the time and is not fully appreciated for it's peculiar properties. The succussed and diluted "water" is then put into it's final available form on pellets or in a liquid and is then used by the patient to counter his/her disease.

How does it work then? It may be used to desensitize a person from exposure to a toxic substance. It may correct a deficiency or more likely an inability on the person's part where they cannot assimilate a much needed mineral. It may counter the life force of a virus or bacteria that has overcome the "Vital Force" pattern of the patient. In other words it can act as an immunization.   Homeopaths call it working with the "Vital Force", which is dynamic or energetic and always changing. Just as we know that the body is always changing and is dynamic we know it is always striving for homeostasis (a balance of health and function or well-being). Somehow the homeopathically prepared remedy has the ability to correct or heal.

Here is a time to consider also the strange characteristic of world wide pandemics or for that matter flus. The Spanish Influenza appeared all over the world at the same time. One explanation is that it was a bird flu. Even that begs questioning. The Spanish Flu casualties have been estimated at seventy million within one year. It seemed to strike everywhere at rapid speed. In India so many died that they could not be burned and were thrown over cliffs which increased the number of "man eating tigers".   In the United States so many died that entre cities lost their police and fire forces. The death spread to every area, even Eskimos were not spared and only one island was said to not have any deaths from that flu. According to actual government statistics, those who used Aspirin relying on allopathic medicine died and on the other hand government statistics show that very few died who used homeopathic medicine.

As flus appear today they really do reach isolated areas and all at the same time. It really is almost an aura, a vibrational force that is behind it. Can we explain this by contagion? I don't think so.

The way homeopathic remedies work, I think, is best explained by an illustration of a computer software program. A software program can be affected by a virus or become corrupted. It can then be corrected by reinstalling or repairing the program. A homeopathic preparation has the ability to do the same and get down to that cellular level. Whether it be ionic or a matter of photons of light, it "speaks the language" of the cells. Unlike herbal preparations that are still in a "gross" state or as pharmaceutically produced synthetic drugs, that do not jive with our natural body cells, homeopathics can reboot the program in the cells with the correct information. In order to do this they must be taken for some time and potency is important too. Realize that our body rebuilds itself approximately every eight months. So, for deeply rooted cellular problems it is usually pretty minimal to take a remedy for that length of time. There is a general rule - one month for every year of a chronic disease condition.

I should emphasize here that synthetic drugs are foreign to our bodies language and the only reason to use them even homeopathically would be to hopefully cancel them out or clear them. This method is referred to as Tautopathy.

Potency is vitally important

Potency revolves around how many times the substance was diluted and sucussed. Diluting a substance is not enough. That will not make a homeopathic remedy. Pounding or succession alone will not produce a homeopathic remedy. A strict set of standards has been established and all is done in absolute sterile environment so that nothing but the remedy is present in the final product. Most remedies are pounded or succussed thousands of time in order to produce the remedy and the exact potency needed can be ordered from the pharmacy. In most cases a series of ever increasing and higher potency over a period of time is carefully prescribed to end the disease symptoms. Hahnemann once said that giving the same potency twice is an insult to the body. I always recommend taking a special prepared liquid and pounding it several times before each dose.

Allopathic drugs have side effects

The results or benefits of homeopathy over allopathic treatment are proven and of great benefit. For one thing allopathic drugs have secondary or "side effects". We are all familiar with them now as commercials are required to warn about them. They are in the PDR (Physician's Desk Reference) and required in leaflet warnings with every prescription you get. Your pharmacist must consult with you and warn you about them. You can look them up online.

The warnings really fall short as they should also tell you this: allopathic drugs cause other diseases. Not so Homeopathic remedies. Homeopathic remedies do not have "secondary effects" as allopathic drugs do. They can cause aggravations which will mean you are experiencing too high a potency (which is why homeopaths start at the lowest possible dose). If it is the wrong remedy for you, you may "prove" the remedy taking on some characteristics of the remedy, that is symptoms that you never had before. They were not the original disease that you had. In this case the effects will soon stop when you stop the remedy or can simply be antidoted with mint, coffee or another remedy. It will not give you a disease as many allopathics do. Some "side effects" of allopathic drugs can be diabetes mellitus or diabetes insipidus. Yes, that "dry mouth" caused by your medication can be much worse than you realize. It can be giving you a full-blown incurable disease. In particular, dry mouth can indicate deep disturbances in the liver, intestines or kidneys caused by the allopathic medicine.

What if I am taking the wrong remedy?

For the most part, if it is the wrong remedy for you, it will not work. That is why it is so important to take a complete case. Homeopaths want to take really good (complete) cases to begin with. They want to analyze in full knowledge of the entire person and their history. They end up dealing a lot with people who are finally fed up with other medicines and who come to them with fairly progressed states. It would be better if they had sought homeopathic treatment earlier. The earlier a person is treated, the faster they will respond to Homeopathic treatment.

One of the greatest examples of this is when a person comes in with Poison Oak. If they take their correct remedy right away I have seen it go away in hours. If they wait days it may take a week or more. If they take it before exposure, (prophylactically like an immunization) they may not get it at all. There are several remedies for Poison Oak. One that worked like a charm for me, I found out, did not work for a friend. Yes, there are several used even for such a simple thing as Poison Oak.

It is frustrating for both the patient and the Homeopath when people want a remedy thrown at them without a proper case taking. Even if you are given the right remedy, it will take a period of time to see it's effect. You don't want to be trying remedy after remedy to see if it's the one. Better to have a good case taken.

To emphasize one last thing regarding the difference between Allopathic and Homeopathic preparations - Allopathic medicines overwhelm the body. They attempt to force it to do something it was never intended to do. They may shut down receptors in a very powerful way or have other violent effects. Many people do not realize that this can be permanent. In fact, many Allopathic "wonder drugs" work this way. In six months the receptors will wither and die. They will never be there again to work in the body as they were made by the "Great Designer" to work. A person generally knows when they have taken an allopathic drug. They can feel it working. A drug may "knock them out" or as it were, "knock them over the head". It also will do them just about as much good. Even coffee, tea, caffeine and that most powerful and abused drug "alcohol" have effects we feel strongly. They overpower the body and it's defenses. They commandeer themselves upon the system, suppressing or forcibly stimulating various bodily hormones or secretions.

On the contrasting side, homeopathic remedies work and all we get is a realization, at some point, that the disease symptoms that we had are finally gone. This will be after a period of time and the time periods can vary according to disease and the person. So, the right homeopathic will manifest as a reduction or elimination of the disease symptoms. During all the treatment until the disease is for sure extinguished, it is good to work with a homeopath.

Potency and how the remedy is taken are extremely important. It is probably one of the foremost reasons self-treatment fails. There is much to know about these things. Sometimes it is necessary to switch to another remedy that can complement or even complete the action of the original remedy. In other words: one remedy may not completely cover or cancel a disease pattern – another one may be needed.

Going back into time

Homeopaths know by many cases that although they will take a case and start with current symptoms, they will eventually be going back into the history of the disease. This may seem strange but older symptoms will reappear in reverse chronological order in chronic cases and may need another remedy or they may just need more time with the current remedy. The Homeopathic Materia Medica and the Homeopathic Repertory must be consulted again. Why go through all this? Because we want a "cure"- a complete and permanent remission of symptoms - not acquisition of another disease by allopathic suppression of symptoms.

Acute and chronic differences

Acutes

Basically, an acute disease is like a flu, cold or one of the epidemics. A person gets it and it progresses to a crisis. You get over it or not. It can result in death if it becomes complicated by bacteria or a viral infection or if a person who is already weak is overwhelmed - is stressed, with other factors. Other factors could be getting not enough sleep, not getting enough vitamins, minerals or Vitamin C during the acute; and as listed above are subjected to further invasion of bacterial or other microbes; severe emotional stresses; a physical trauma on top of the disease; exposure to cold or heat that is extreme; or any other thing that overwhelms the body's immune system.

When an acute becomes a chronic

Chicken pox is an acute but can progress into other stages. Diseases much later in life can be the result of that case of chicken pox that you had as a child. On the other hand, measles is an acute and amazingly, although people get over it, there is evidence that it can provide long term immune benefits. When a person gets an acute it should provide life-long immunity from that particular strain of pathogen.

Vaccinations
This is not the case with vaccinations. The situation is not that the principle of vaccination does not work, as it is actually a Homeopathic concept or Isopathic, but it has been corrupted by adding adjuvants as well as contamination of other live organism, as well as by using live organisms. This is dangerous and not necessary. <u>Also, the method of delivery through intra-muscular injections which go straight into the bloodstream and can induce anaphylactic shock followed by death or brain damage is unnecessary and deadly.</u> The history of the polio vaccination shows how great the danger of contamination has been by organisms other than the ingredients of said so-called vaccinations. An entire

generation has, in effect, been given cancer. See the book "Dr Mary's Monkey" by Edward T. Haslam

In the case of the naturally occurring process of acquiring resistance, we do see exceptions to this and when a person gets the same acute over and over we look to an underlying "miasmatic" obstacle. A study of miasms is deep but is similar to what we would call genetic predisposition, but not exactly the same.

There are definitely lingering recurrences seen in whooping cough in many cases, but there are also remedies that are known to cancel out these particular after effects and in actuality continue to work to extinguish the full expression of that disease. It can take more than one remedy to completely put out the fires of a disease . Diseases are really more complex than anyone has been able to fully study. Whooping cough is one of these cases. The persistent and recurrent expressions of whooping cough reveal that the disease is still active in the symptoms that it pushes out to be presented in the patient. In this case an acute has become a chronic.

There are cases of people who will get the same acute over and over, it seems that they cannot develop a true resistance to a disease. Homeopaths look to understand this as a "miasmatic" obstacle. They have good ways to deal with this and in my opinion you can't completely heal the person without addressing the miasmatic component in the person. Once the miasmatic component is dealt with, there is a removal of the miasmatic blockage, freeing up the way so that the effective remedy for the recurring acute or chronic can be reintroduced with success.

More on what appears to be an acute

One symptom could be when a person gets colds all the time. Some people are constantly having bronchitis or are hoarse. Another could be having heartburn all the time. Infections or wounds that do not heal is another one. These all show an underlying condition. In other words what might look like a recurring acute is really a chronic that has peaked or flared up repeatedly showing a condition that the body cannot overcome by itself. It will do no good to use a suppressive allopathic method but the true origin of the condition must be dealt with. Even a medical doctor recognizes this when a person is really exhibiting signs of diabetes.

The fact that most all people are on their way to developing a chronic disease shows the necessity of having a most meticulous case taking by the homeopath before trying to analyze the patient, even for an acute. It is best to have all the information possible on hand in order to make the best choices for a patient. If the homeopath is not aware of everything in the patient's history, the wrong conclusion can be drawn. The remedy selection may be inadequate and real treatment is delayed. This can be frustrating for the patient and the homeopath.

In regards to knowing everything about a patient, I can give two examples where complete information was not given and the right remedy was not given. One involves a man who was bitten by a rabid dog and then given the anti-rabies shots. This was extremely important information for the homeopath to have, but was never given. Another one, that happens a lot is people will not give information that they have had a venereal disease. Or as they say today – an S.T.D. Usually this will be admitted later in the case. Patients should know that there is no judgment by the homeopath. They just want to get it all in the initial case taking and give the patient the best chance of recovering.

Understanding chronic disease

A chronic disease is basically one that the body cannot get rid of by it's own usual efforts. It can manifest in a multitude of ways on any part of the body. When I say by it's own efforts, in fact, it seems at times to sabotage itself. <u>The body may be treating this chronic condition as if it were an acute because it does not have all the tools and knowledge to deal with a manifestation.</u> I would like to give you an example. In the case of cholera, the body will eliminate to the point of complete dehydration and death. The pathogen is so noxious to the body it only knows that it must get rid of the toxin. In most cases of diarrhea it would be wrong to allopathically suppress or stop diarrhea with medications but in the case of cholera something must be done or the very intrinsic defense system of the body will cause death. Yes, the body can be "dumb" at times. As I mentioned earlier , allopathic or suppressive methods may be necessary and have their place and can be life-saving. But is that all that can be done? Is an allopathic solution all that there is? Isopathic treatment through immunization is one solution but is not always possible. The homeopathic solution would be to use a substance that manifests the same symptoms as the disease. This has been done in the form of various homeopathic remedies and has worked better than allopathic suppression. The fact is that giving a "remedy" with the same symptoms as that stage of that acute has worked to stop the progress of an acute. Suppression is not always a good idea especially if a homeopathic works. If not, then loss of fluids and continuous diarrhea must be stopped.

But what about true chronic conditions? We can see that chronic conditions are by far the most debilitating to our life. Yes, we usually get over that flu or even the measles and other conditions but what about arthritis, mental illness, heart disease, kidney disease and other chronic diseases? Why is our body not able to fend off these diseases?

The beginnings of a chronic disease building up can be subtle. When it is still at this level, in a more subtle state, is the best time to extinguish it with Homeopathic methods, that is, in it's early stages. Homeopathy works best at these early or first stages when it is still on an energetic level, just as homeopathy is an energetic level of healing. Homeopathy considers that disease begins as an "untunement" of the "Vital Force". While people think that their yearly physical and bloodwork will warn them of impending disease, homeopathic symptoms are much more revealing about what is to come in what has been studied and revealed as "constitutional patterns".   By strengthening the person's body and not by attacking a "disease" per-se many cures have come about. Indeed, chronic disease has much to do with the constitution of the person.

Dreams and homeopathy

 Most interesting to me are that dreams can warn us of or tell us much about what processes are going on in our own body. Not in the occult sense but as a natural result of what is going on in the body. Dreams have much to do with the emotional

body. I believe that dreams are the point, the meeting ground for the physical and the emotional body.
They are really two worlds. The place where dreams and the "real" physical world meet to try to make sense of things or reconcile.

Dreams can be the revealer of what is going on. In harmony with this, people have told me that their dreams change with the remedy or if they are not dreaming, they will start to dream. Nightmares will stop or modify. I like for patients to keep a note of their dreams as it is very helpful to stay on course with their remedy decisions. I have had some very interesting experiences with patients and dreams. Of course, I am very aware of the effect of homeopathic remedies and the sleep state.

In actuality Dreams can be the revealer of what is going on. In harmony with this, people have told me that their dreams change with the remedy or if they are not dreaming, they will start to dream. Nightmares will stop or modify. I like for patients to keep a note of their dreams as it is very helpful to stay on course with their remedy decisions. I have had some very interesting experiences with patients and dreams. Of course, I am very aware of the effect of homeopathic remedies and the sleep state.

The Emotional body is who we are

Many in the Homeopathic field know that all illness begins in the emotional body. Perhaps more correctly, it could be said that the incongruity between the two worlds, the disparity, the lack of harmony, or the lack of resolution we find between the dreams in our heart and the way life goes, cause disease.

Let me enlarge on this. A child realizes that she wants to be a dancer or a singer. It is the dream of her heart. Instead of encouragement, her parents laugh and don't take her seriously. She is burdened with every kind of drudgery so that she never has time to pursue her heart's desire. Then the other people she has come to consider as an authority figure in her life tell her that her desire to be a singer and a dancer is selfish and furthermore that she has to choose between God and her selfish desires. Although she struggles with this and even makes sacrifices to take lessons and pursue it, the authority figures and her parents win out, making it impossible for her to find her happiness with her natural God-given gifts. She faces a life torn apart between divergent allegiances and can never reconcile them. It takes a life time of psychological warfare within to come to terms and in the meantime, her body falters. She suffers from intractable insomnia, weakness and her immune system is always compromised. A rare occurrence. I think not. It is really a complexity that she found out many suffer from. Yes, "dreams die hard". All of these things Homeopathy takes note of. Every remedy has a mental profile, most have a dream profile or lack of dreaming. Indeed, when remedies are "proven" any action on any part of the body or psyche, and every sensation is faithfully recorded as a science. "Provings" are done on groups of people and are compared but each individual study is also noted separately.

Illness begins In the emotional body

I can think of one very big example of how a "disease" began in the "spirit" or the emotional body and then progressed into a chronic disease and finally led to the ultimate death of a woman. This is a true story about someone I knew well. I do not use her real name.

Case

Hazel was molested as a young girl. It was a bad case of molestation as she actually contracted syphilis from her molester. Later she passed Syphilis on to her children as well. The emotional pain she felt was unbearable and she handled her rage and sense of violation by binging on food. Whether she had bulimia I am not certain, but she told me she reached close to 400 pounds.   What kind of psychiatric help she got I am not certain as she was not a homeopathic client of mine. The fact is she was not able to get her weight down and carried it for many years. Eventually the allopathic community of medical care offered her the procedure where they remove a good part of the small intestine. She had this done and did lose weight. Another "triumph" for the Allopathic doctors although it has, the last time I checked, a 25% mortality rate. A rather risky surgery but we know how desperate people are to lose weight, but at what cost? The "triumph" was bitter though as the "after effects" progressed. After this her kidneys failed. This is a frequent occurrence after this "medical procedure". Her brother was good enough to donate one of his kidneys to his sister. A noble act, but of course that affected his health adversely. Truly, he gave his life. Please don't believe it when the doctors tell you that you only need one kidney or that you don't need your gall bladder or appendix or tonsils.   I met her at this point and it wasn't long before her one donated kidney failed. She began the difficult life on the dialysis machine. Now she was totally reliant on kidney dialysis. A costly treatment that she could not afford without funding.

Not life at it's best. As the few years that I knew her went by I watched her turn into an emaciated "concentration camp victim look". Finally, they could no longer find a place to insert the dialysis and they just shunted it straight into her heart. She clung to me for massage as long as possible. I know what this is about as people who are in severe pain seek to compensate the state of always being in pain with something that will give their poor bodies a state of pleasure. When she made the last appointment, I looked at her and said, "Are you sure you want another appointment?" She wanted massage more than anything. She loved the essential oils and credited them with preserving her life. Even other medical workers could not understand why she was still alive. She made the appointment, but she was deceased before I saw her again.

The reason I bring up this very sad but true story is to show the stages of treatment she got from allopathic medicine. Her "illness" truly began in her emotional body. First, if she received psychiatric drugs they blocked her ability to process trauma on an emotional basis, which is what she needed, this again was detrimental.   Psychiatric drugs in their allopathic pharmacy have no ability to negotiate the higher levels of consciousness on a cellular level as the homeopathic preparations have proven to do.   Homeopathic pharmacy works on a higher level than the material.   If she received counseling that is good, but it has proven again and again not to be completely effective.   When a person goes over and over the same trauma it reinforces it in the memory and I think it is like making a rut in the brain. I have seen people who after 10 years of talk therapy were no better, have you? (I recommend REM therapy) Later, her desperate choice to have her small intestines drastically reduced in surgery led to an even more dire situation – the shut-down of her kidneys – a vital organ.

This is only a typical case.   Once in the clutches of the medical establish, one dire choice gives birth to the next. It even affects another's health being called upon to donate organs and has created an abomination called the organ industry becoming truly the most macabre and evil enterprises the world has ever seen. In spite of the propaganda put out by the medical establishment, life with any kind of transplant, with anti-rejection drugs and eventual death from that is not desirable. It is much more complicated and painful than many even begin to comprehend. At the expense of unimaginable suffering the medical industry makes obscene billions from their obscene procedures.

So, what began in the "emotional body" with Hazel after being victimized became an emotional monster, producing a disease that was treated allopathically, developing into a more severe disease and then organ failure and reliance on very expensive treatment that she could not avoid if she wanted to live another week. It also impacted and cut short the life of her brother. Her emotional trauma was never resolved. I saw the pain in her life was day after day, after day.

Surely, we want something better than this. This would be an example of a disease that began in the emotional body. I would like to believe that if she had been treated from the beginning with the appropriate homeopathic treatment she would never have developed her impossible weight problem. If she had sought out Homeopathic treatment, she would not have been further complicated by the allopathic answer - surgery, transplant and resulting kidney failure. What a futility! None of which got to the heart of the matter. There are many examples which are not so clear, but never the less upon close examination began after emotional trauma that a person did not recover from.

Other causes of chronic disease

Another cause of chronic disease are accidents of one type or another, whether it be blunt trauma or chemical exposure, radiation, etc. which are all outside forces that can induce a disease that will be chronic. In all these cases, emotional shock is very much a part of the profile and needs to be addressed with homeopathy. Yes, people really notice the help Homeopathics provide for these things. I have experienced it and others report their progress to me as well. Do not let anyone tell you there are - "no case histories". That is ridiculous! Homeopathy provides hundreds of thousands of case histories for a multitude of diseases and their origins in the emotional body.

While Allopathic emergency care may be necessary, and in fact offers life saving techniques, Allopathic medicines have failed deplorably for chronic disease. Patients unhappy or disillusioned with what they are getting for their chronic or unexplained disease seek out many forms of alternative care. They often do this looking for herbal or even concentrated forms of chemicals with such a lack of understanding that they only compound their issues. If it helped Aunt Thelma then it must be going to help them. All the while Homeopathic resources are used the same with little benefits. People use "combination remedies" and may get an initial response but then find it stops. They know little about how Homeopathic theory works.

Doctors and those in the medical field will criticize. The fact is death is eventually inevitable for all of us. However, people feel better and can still function well in many cases with homeopathy and other alternative care. There are a multitude of cases where disease symptoms were completely extinguished by homeopathy and never did return. There are cases of people of cancer who where death was expected in days who had complete "remissions" for unknown reasons.

Those interested in homeopathy will find it a vast field that can be overwhelming at times. It is a fascinating study for those who have that inclination.

I hope I have enlightened the reader so that the true experience of homeopathy can be realized.
It is best to work with a Homeopath who has had training in Classical Homeopathy. There are approximately seven thousand remedies available to Homeopaths. They can be poly-crests which cover some very big patterns in people or they can be very specific, working on only one area. Remedies have an affinity for nerves, or muscles, mucous linings, different organs, etc.. Remedies have affinity for specific nerves, organs and bones. Remedies identify with specific pains, lesions and organisms. It is a very complex study and even then homeopaths use computers to help analyze each case. Another reason to seek out a good homeopath is the fact that it is very difficult to treat oneself. The emotional state is primary for each remedy. Some people don't realize that they are hysterical! Some people don't want to admit that they are overflowing with hatred or that the grief they carry is still with them and destroying them. The point is, it is difficult to be objective about one's

own self and even a child or loved one that you are emotionally entangled with.

Today, there are homeopaths who have trained in special fields in homeopathy. Most all of these should have had training in Classical Homeopathy. One example of a special field would be those who practice CEASE therapy which is especially geared for children with Autism Spectrum Disorders. They have had specialized training for that. Although many have developed protocols for such cases, the alert Homeopath should always be aware of symptoms that call for a modification of their treatment that supports the individual constitution of the person.

I have a thirty-two page intake form and have spent many hours initially with patients. Each case is like solving a mystery. It is like Sherlock Holmes is on the case. In homeopathy you must be alert and keep your mind open. It is important to not presume or pigeon-hole people. Every case sends me to research. I find I cannot leave the case till I come close to breaking it. I get up in the night and I am reading or on the computer researching.

Homeopathy, in some ways, is simple and at the same time can be complex to take care of. Chronic cases are more complex. Cases can be layered. This is especially true with the cases that have been treated with a lot of allopathic medications.

People are dynamic, changing, living beings. It is very important to work with a homeopath and not just try to figure it out on your own. It is difficult to be objective about ourselves. Also, there are various guiding rules that homeopaths follow to obtain the best results. It is not easy sometimes to decide where to start! Also homeopaths have computer programs that help to analyze remedies and their properties and their value for various conditions. Some remedies are better than others for some manifestations and have concomitant properties that are either in agreement with treatment or may not be desirable for the complete picture.

Some of these computer programs cost thousands of dollars and buying one is not warranted unless one wants to pursue a professional Homeopathic career. More than monetary concerns, Homeopathic training takes four to five years for most people and requires a high level of patience for endless hours of study. Actually, until you reach a certain level you may fear you will lose your mind with all that you must study and put together!

Another negative aspect of self diagnosis is that when a person does not feel well they are just not in the state to do research and analyze their situation very well. They are, as I say, chasing their own tail. They see a description of every disease in themselves. That is not how a serious subject is studied! Let someone look after you!

I hope that this encourages everyone to seek out a professional Homeopath and also to increase their own knowledge about Homeopathy. In my many hours of study and research I have no doubt that the foundation of homeopathy is divine in origin. It is a system that has been there all along and may have been practiced in it's totality in the ancient past when life expectancy was far longer. It is a science only recent in it's discovery and much is yet to be learned and much to be organized to improve it's use. I am in the process of organizing a lot of information that is scattered from many sources.

More than I can prove to some, let me say from my heart that I have gone through a lot to present the experience I suffered and the curative powers in Homeopathy. I desire nothing but what is true and best for you. It is available and it is real in Homeopathy. Please experience it for yourself.

Books by Martha Y. Wright

The Mermaid of the Kyle-of-Localsh & Journey to Skye: a story for the child & a story for the parents

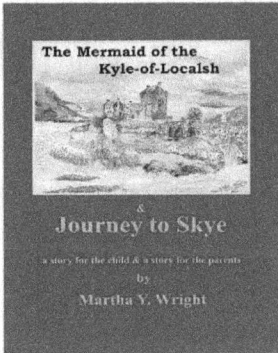

a tale followed by a true story

@ amazon.com

https://www.amazon.com/s/ref=nb_
sb_noss?url=search-alias%3Daps&field-keywords=
The+Mermaid+of+the+Kyle-of-Localsh+%26+Journey+to+Skye

How the Movies Saved My Life & Other Themes 1961 – 2017

On Amazon.com

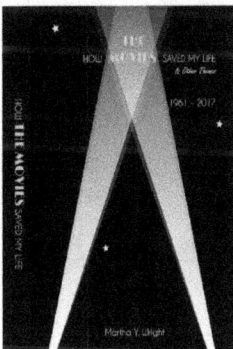

How the Movies Saved My Life

& Other Themes 1961 - 2017

by

Martha Y. Wright

www.amazon.com/s/ref=hb_sb_noss?url
=search-alias%3Daps&field-Keywords=
How+the+Movies++Saved+my+Life

Lyme Disease: How I Beat It

@Amazon.com

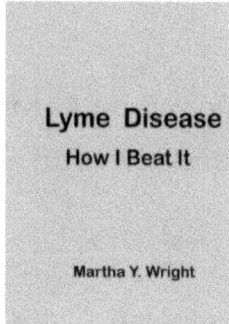

https://www.amazon.com/Lyme-Disease-How-I-
Beat/dp/0692102825/ref=sr_1_fkmr0_4?s=books&ie=UTF8&
qid=1535928525&sr=1-4-
fkmr0&keywords=Ly%2Cme+disease+how+I+beat+it+by+Mar
tha+Wrught

Contact Martha Y. Wright @

www.homeopathicliving.com

Books of interest

Narayana-verlag.com   has many homeopathic publications

Doctor Mary's Monkey   by Edward T. Haslam

www.ingramcontent.com/pod-product-compliance
Lightning Source LLC
Chambersburg PA
CBHW070814280326
41934CB00012B/3191